Air Fryer Quick Recipes

Don't Miss These Quick and Easy Recipes to
Make Incredible Air Fryer Appetizers

Eva Sheppard

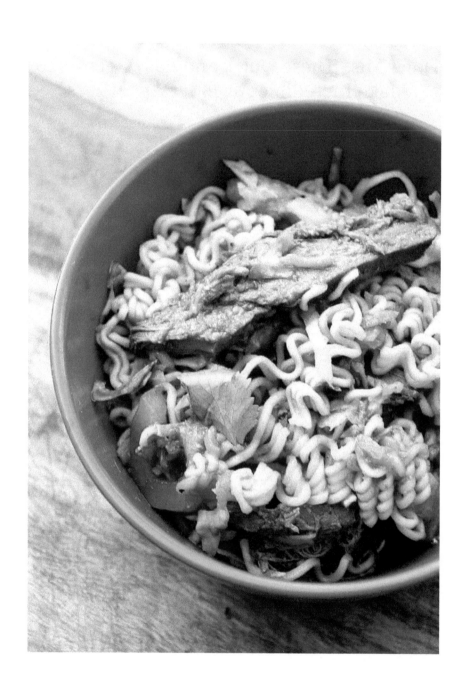

or implied. Readers acknowledge that the author is not engaging in the rendering of legal, financial, medical or professional advice. The content within this book has been derived from various sources. Please consult a licensed professional before attempting any techniques outlined in this book.

By reading this document, the reader agrees that under no circumstances is the author responsible for any losses, direct or indirect, which are incurred as a result of the use of information contained within this document, including, but not limited to, — errors, omissions, or inaccuracies.

TABLE OF CONTENT

Chinese Cabbage & Beef Bowls

Preparation Time: 22 minutes

Servings: 5

Ingredients:

- Sirloin steak-1/2 pound -cut into strips
- Soy sauce-1 tbsp
- Olive oil-1 tbsp
- Salt and black pepper to taste
- Green cabbage-2 cups -shredded
- Green onions-2 -chopped
- Yellow bell pepper-1 -chopped
- Garlic cloves-2 -minced

Directions:

1. Pick a pan that fits your air fryer and mix the cabbage, salt, pepper, and oil.

2. After tossing well, put the pan in your air fryer and cook at 370 o F for 4 minutes.

3. Combine the steak, green onions, bell peppers, soy sauce, and garlic.

4. Toss and cover to cook for another 6 minutes.

5. Divide into bowls and serve.

Nutrition Values:

calories 262, fat 9, fiber 8, carbs 14, protein 11

Pudding With Veggies

Preparation Time: 43 minutes

Servings: 7

Ingredients:

- Butter-1 tbsp -softened
- Yellow onion-1 -chopped
- Corn-2 cups
- Celery-1/4 cup -chopped
- Thyme-1 tsp -chopped
- Red bell peppers-2 -chopped
- Garlic-2 tsp -minced
- Heavy cream-1/2 cup
- Salt and black pepper to taste
- Milk-1-1/2 cups
- Bread-3 cups -cubed
- Eggs-3 -whisked
- Cheddar cheese-4 tbsps -grated

Directions:

1. Butter to grease a baking dish that fits your air fryer.

2. Mix all other ingredients except the cheddar cheese.

3. After tossing well, sprinkle the cheese all over.

4. Place the dish in the fryer, and cook at 360 o F for 30 minutes.

5. Divide between plates, serve, and enjoy.

Nutrition Values:

calories 286, fat 10, fiber 2, carbs 16, protein 11

Lunch of Coconut Zucchini

Preparation Time: 23 minutes

Servings: 9

Ingredients:

- Veggie stock-1 cup
- Zucchinis-8 -cut in medium wedges
- Coconut cream-1 cup
- Soy sauce-1 tbsp
- Rosemary-1/4 tsp -dried
- Olive oil-2 tbsps
- Yellow onions-2 -chopped
- Salt and black pepper to taste
- Thyme-1/4 tsp -dried
- Basil-1/2 tsp -chopped

Directions:

1. Pick a pan that fits your air fryer and grease it with the oil.

2. Combine all other ingredients to the pan.

3. After tossing, place the pan in the fryer.

4. Cook at 360 o F for 16 minutes.

5. Divide the mix between plates, serve, and enjoy.

Nutrition Values:

calories 181, fat 4, fiber 4, carbs 10, protein 5

Simple Kale and Mushroom Chicken Mix

Preparation Time: 27 minutes

Servings: 7

Ingredients:

- A bunch of kale -torn
- Chicken stock-2 tbsps
- Salt and black pepper to taste
- Tomato sauce-1/4 cup
- Shiitake mushrooms-1-1/2 cups -roughly sliced
- Chicken breast-1 cup -skinless, boneless, cooked and shredded

Directions:

1. Pick a pan that fits your air fryer and mix all ingredients.

2. Toss and then put the pan in the fryer.

3. Cook at 350 o F for 20 minutes.

4. Divide between plates and serve.

14

Nutrition Values:

calories 210, fat 7, fiber 2, carbs 14, protein 5

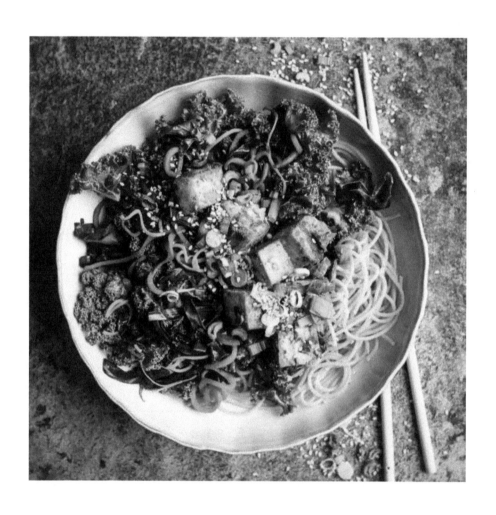

Chicken Casserole With Beans

Preparation Time: 33 minutes

Servings: 7

Ingredients:

- Chicken breast-3 cups -skinless, boneless, cooked and shredded
- Cilantro-1/2 cup -chopped
- Canned black beans-24 ounces -drained and rinsed
- Mozzarella cheese-3 cups -shredded
- Kale leaves-6 -chopped
- Salsa-2 cups
- Green onions-1/2 cup -chopped
- A drizzle of olive oil
- Cumin-2 tsp -ground
- Chili powder-2 tsp
- Garlic powder-1 tbsp

Directions:

1. Take a baking dish that fits your air fryer and grease it with the oil.

2. Add all other ingredients except the cheese to the baking dish.

3. Then sprinkle the cheese all over and place the dish in the air fryer.

4. Cook at 350 o F for 20 minutes.

5. Divide between plates, serve, and enjoy!

Nutrition Values:

calories 285, fat 12, fiber 6, carbs 22, protein 15

Japanese Style Chicken

Preparation Time: 18 Minutes

Servings: 2

Ingredients:

- 2 chicken thighs; skinless and boneless
- 1/8 cup sake
- 1/2 tsp. sesame oil
- 1/8 cup water
- 2 ginger slices; chopped
- 3 garlic cloves; minced
- 1/4 cup soy sauce
- 1/4 cup mirin
- 2 tbsp. sugar
- 1 tbsp. cornstarch mixed with 2 tbsp. water
- Sesame seeds for serving

Directions:

1. In a bowl; mix chicken thighs with ginger, garlic, soy sauce, mirin, sake, oil, water,

sugar and cornstarch; toss well, transfer to preheated air fryer and cook at 360 °F, for 8 minutes. Divide among plates; sprinkle sesame seeds on top and serve with a side salad for lunch.

Nutrition Values: Calories: 300; Fat: 7; Fiber: 9; Carbs: 17; Protein: 10

Chicken Pie Recipe

Preparation Time: 29 Minutes

Servings: 4

Ingredients:

- 2 chicken thighs; boneless, skinless and cubed
- 1 carrot; chopped
- 1 tsp. Worcestershire sauce
- 1 tbsp. flour
- 1 tbsp. milk
- 2 puff pastry sheets
- 1 tbsp. butter; melted
- 1 yellow onion; chopped
- 2 potatoes; chopped
- 2 mushrooms; chopped
- 1 tsp. soy sauce
- Salt and black pepper to the taste
- 1 tsp. Italian seasoning
- 1/2 tsp. garlic powder

Directions:

2. Heat up a pan over medium high heat, add potatoes, carrots and onion; stir and cook for 2 minutes.

3. Add chicken and mushrooms, salt, soy sauce, pepper, Italian seasoning, garlic powder, Worcestershire sauce, flour and milk; stir really well and take off heat.

4. Place 1 puff pastry sheet on the bottom of your air fryer's pan and trim edge excess.

5. Add chicken mix, top with the other puff pastry sheet; trim excess as well and brush pie with butter.

6. Place in your air fryer and cook at 360 °F, for 6 minutes. Leave pie to cool down; slice and serve for breakfast.

Nutrition Values: Calories: 300; Fat: 5; Fiber: 7; Carbs: 14; Protein: 7

Chicken Fajitas

Preparation Time: 20 Minutes

Servings: 4

Ingredients:

- 1 lb. chicken breasts; cut into strips
- 1 tsp. garlic powder
- 1/4 tsp. cumin; ground
- 1/2 tsp. chili powder
- 1 green bell pepper; sliced
- 1 yellow onion; chopped.
- 1 tbsp. lime juice
- 1/4 tsp. coriander; ground
- 1 red bell pepper; sliced
- Salt and black pepper to the taste
- Cooking spray
- 4 tortillas; warmed up
- Salsa for serving
- 1 cup lettuce leaves; torn for serving
- Sour cream for serving

Directions:

1. In a bowl; mix chicken with garlic powder, cumin, chili, salt, pepper, coriander, lime juice, red bell pepper, green bell pepper and onion; toss, leave aside for 10 minutes, transfer to your air fryer and drizzle some cooking spray all over.

2. Toss and cook at 400 °F, for 10 minutes. Arrange tortillas on a working surface, divide chicken mix, also add salsa, sour cream and lettuce; wrap and serve for lunch.

Nutrition Values: Calories: 317; Fat: 6; Fiber: 8; Carbs: 14; Protein: 4

Lentils Fritters

Preparation Time: 20 Minutes

Servings: 2

Ingredients:

- 1 cup yellow lentils; soaked in water for 1 hour and drained
- 1 hot chili pepper; chopped.
- 1-inch ginger piece; grated
- 1/2 tsp. turmeric powder
- 1 tsp. garam masala
- 1 tsp. baking powder
- 2 tsp. olive oil
- 1/3 cup water
- 1/2 cup cilantro; chopped
- 1 ½ cup spinach; chopped
- 4 garlic cloves; minced
- 3/4 cup red onion; chopped
- Salt and black pepper to the taste
- Mint chutney for serving

Directions:

1. In your blender; mix lentils with chili pepper, ginger, turmeric, garam masala, baking powder, salt, pepper, olive oil, water, cilantro, spinach, onion and garlic, blend well and shape medium balls out of this mix.

2. Place them all in your preheated air fryer at 400 °F and cook for 10 minutes. Serve your veggie fritters with a side salad for lunch.

Nutrition Values: Calories: 142; Fat: 2; Fiber: 8; Carbs: 12; Protein: 4

Corn Casserole Recipe

Preparation Time: 25 Minutes

Servings: 4

Ingredients:

- 2 cups corn

- 1/2 cup light cream

- 1/2 cup Swiss cheese; grated

- 2 tbsp. butter

- 3 tbsp. flour

- 1 egg

- 1/4 cup milk

- Salt and black pepper to the taste

- Cooking spray

Directions:

1. In a bowl; mix corn with flour, egg, milk, light cream, cheese, salt, pepper and butter and stir well.

2. Grease your air fryer's pan with cooking spray, pour cream mix; spread and cook at

320 °F, for 15 minutes. Serve warm for lunch.

Nutrition Values: Calories: 281; Fat: 7; Fiber: 8; Carbs: 9; Protein: 6

Fish And Kettle Chips

Preparation Time: 22 Minutes

Servings: 2

Ingredients:

- 2 medium cod fillets; skinless and boneless
- 1/4 cup buttermilk
- 3 cups kettle chips; cooked
- Salt and black pepper to the taste

Directions:

1. In a bowl mix fish with salt, pepper and buttermilk; toss and leave aside for 5 minutes.

2. Put chips in your food processor, crush them and spread them on a plate.

3. Add fish and press well on all sides.

4. Transfer fish to your air fryer's basket and cook at 400 °F, for 12 minutes. Serve hot for lunch.

Nutrition Values: Calories: 271; Fat: 7; Fiber: 9; Carbs: 14; Protein: 4

Steak and Cabbage

Preparation Time: 20 Minutes

Servings: 4

Ingredients:

- 1/2 lb. sirloin steak; cut into strips
- 2 green onions; chopped.
- 2 garlic cloves; minced
- 2 tsp. cornstarch
- 1 tbsp. peanut oil
- 2 cups green cabbage; chopped
- 1 yellow bell pepper; chopped
- Salt and black pepper to the taste

Directions:

1. In a bowl; mix cabbage with salt, pepper and peanut oil; toss, transfer to air fryer's basket, cook at 370 °F, for 4 minutes and transfer to a bowl.

2. Add steak strips to your air fryer; also add green onions, bell pepper, garlic, salt and

pepper, toss and cook for 5 minutes. Add over cabbage; toss, divide among plates and serve for lunch.

Nutrition Values: Calories: 282; Fat: 6; Fiber: 8; Carbs: 14; Protein: 6

Chicken Wings

Preparation Time: 55 Minutes

Servings: 4

Ingredients:

- 3 lbs. chicken wings
- 3/4 cup potato starch
- 1 tsp. lemon juice
- 1/2 cup butter
- 1 tbsp. old bay seasoning
- Lemon wedges for serving

Directions:

1. In a bowl; mix starch with old bay seasoning and chicken wings and toss well.

2. Place chicken wings in your air fryer's basket and cook them at 360 °F, for 35 minutes shaking the fryer from time to time.

3. Increase temperature to 400 degrees F; cook chicken wings for 10 minutes more and divide them on plates.

4. Heat up a pan over medium heat; add butter and melt it.

5. Add lemon juice; stir well, take off heat and drizzle over chicken wings. Serve them for lunch with lemon wedges on the side.

Nutrition Values: Calories: 271; Fat: 6; Fiber: 8; Carbs: 18; Protein: 18

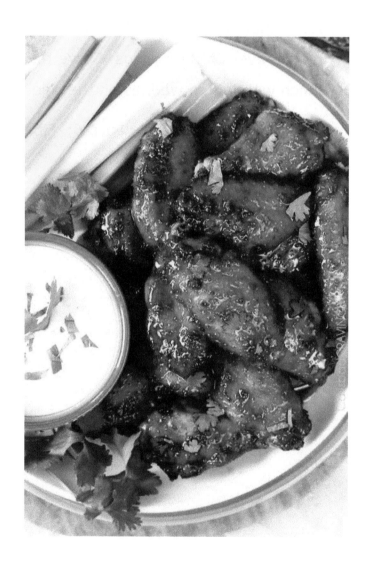

Shrimp Croquettes

Preparation Time: 18 Minutes

Servings: 4

Ingredients:

- 2/3 lb. shrimp; cooked; peeled; deveined and chopped.
- 1 ½ cups bread crumbs
- 1 egg; whisked
- 2 tbsp. olive oil
- 2 tbsp. lemon juice
- 3 green onions; chopped.
- 1/2 tsp. basil; dried
- Salt and black pepper to the taste

Directions:

1. In a bowl; mix half of the bread crumbs with egg and lemon juice and stir well.

2. Add green onions, basil, salt, pepper and shrimp and stir really well.

3. In a separate bowl; mix the rest of the bread crumbs with the oil and toss well.

4. Shape round balls out of shrimp mix, dredge them in bread crumbs; place them in preheated air fryer and cook the for 8 minutes at 400 degrees F. Serve them with a dip for lunch.

Nutrition Values: Calories: 142; Fat: 4; Fiber: 6; Carbs: 9; Protein: 4

Shrimp Pancake

Preparation Time: 20 Minutes

Servings: 2

Ingredients:

- 1 cup small shrimp; peeled and deveined
- 1 tbsp. butter
- 3 eggs; whisked
- 1/2 cup flour
- 1/2 cup milk
- 1 cup salsa

Directions:

1. Preheat your air fryer at 400 degrees F; add fryer's pan, add 1 tbsp. butter and melt it.

2. In a bowl; mix eggs with flour and milk, whisk well and pour into air fryer's pan, spread, cook at 350 degrees for 12 minutes and transfer to a plate. In a bowl; mix shrimp with salsa; stir and serve your pancake with this on the side.

Nutrition Values: Calories: 200; Fat: 6; Fiber: 8; Carbs: 12; Protein: 4

Pork and Potatoes Recipe

Preparation Time: 35 Minutes

Servings: 2

Ingredients:

- 2 lbs. pork loin
- 2 red potatoes; cut into medium wedges
- 1/2 tsp. garlic powder
- 1/2 tsp. red pepper flakes
- 1 tsp. parsley; dried
- A drizzle of balsamic vinegar
- Salt and black pepper to the taste

Directions:

1. In your air fryer's pan; mix pork with potatoes, salt, pepper, garlic powder, pepper flakes, parsley and vinegar; toss and cook at 390 °F, for 25 minutes. Slice pork, divide it and potatoes on plates and serve for lunch.

Nutrition Values: Calories: 400; Fat: 15; Fiber: 7; Carbs: 27; Protein: 20

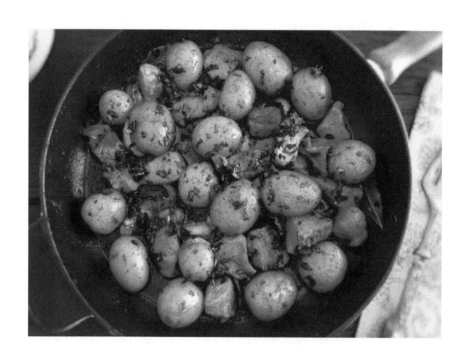

Lunch Pizzas

Preparation Time: 17 Minutes

Servings: 4

Ingredients:

- 3/4 cup pizza sauce

- 2 green onions; chopped

- 2 cup mozzarella; grated

- 4 pitas

- 1 tbsp. olive oil

- 4 oz. jarred mushrooms; sliced

- 1/2 tsp. basil; dried

- 1 cup grape tomatoes; sliced

Directions:

1. Spread pizza sauce on each pita bread; sprinkle green onions and basil, divide mushrooms and top with cheese.

2. Arrange pita pizzas in your air fryer and cook them at 400 °F, for 7 minutes. Top

each pizza with tomato slices; divide among plates and serve.

Nutrition Values: Calories: 200; Fat: 4; Fiber: 6; Carbs: 7; Protein: 3

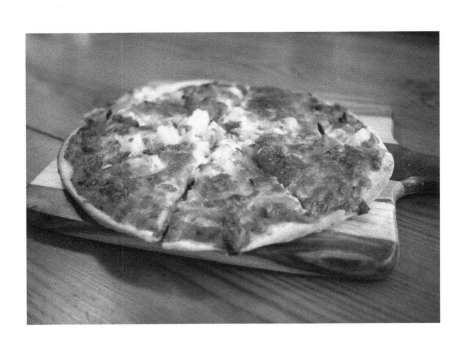

Asparagus and Salmon

Preparation Time: 33 Minutes

Servings: 4

Ingredients:

- 1 lb. asparagus; trimmed
- 1 tbsp. olive oil
- A pinch of sweet paprika
- A pinch of garlic powder
- A pinch of cayenne pepper
- 1 red bell pepper; cut into halves
- 4 oz. smoked salmon
- Salt and black pepper to the taste

Directions:

1. Put asparagus spears and bell pepper on a lined baking sheet that fits your air fryer; add salt, pepper, garlic powder, paprika, olive oil, cayenne pepper, toss to coat, introduce in the fryer; cook at 390 °F, for 8 minutes, flip and cook for 8 minutes more.

Add salmon, cook for 5 minutes more; divide everything on plates and serve.

Nutrition Values: Calories: 90; Fat: 1; Fiber: 1; Carbs: 1.2; Protein: 4

Dill and Scallops

Preparation Time: 15 Minutes

Servings: 4

Ingredients:

- 1 lb. sea scallops; debearded
- 1 tsp. dill; chopped.
- 2 tsp. olive oil
- 1 tbsp. lemon juice
- Salt and black pepper to the taste

Directions:

1. In your air fryer, mix scallops with dill, oil, salt, pepper and lemon juice; cover and cook at 360 °F, for 5 minutes. Discard unopened ones, divide scallops and dill sauce on plates and serve for lunch.

Nutrition Values: Calories: 152; Fat: 4; Fiber: 7; Carbs: 19; Protein: 4

95. Beef Cubes

Preparation Time: 22 Minutes

Servings: 4

Ingredients:

- 1 lb. sirloin; cubed

- 16 oz. jarred pasta sauce

- 1 ½ cups bread crumbs

- 1/2 tsp. marjoram; dried

- 2 tbsp. olive oil

- White rice; already cooked for serving

Directions:

1. In a bowl; mix beef cubes with pasta sauce and toss well.

2. In another bowl; mix bread crumbs with marjoram and oil and stir well.

3. Dip beef cubes in this mix, place them in your air fryer and cook at 360 °F, for 12 minutes. Divide among plates and serve with white rice on the side.

Nutrition Values: Calories: 271; Fat: 6; Fiber: 9; Carbs: 18; Protein: 12

Zucchini and Tuna Tortillas

Preparation Time: 20 Minutes

Servings: 4

Ingredients:

- 1 cup zucchini; shredded
- 1/3 cup mayonnaise
- 2 tbsp. mustard
- 4 corn tortillas
- 4 tbsp. butter; soft
- 6 oz. canned tuna; drained
- 1 cup cheddar cheese; grated

Directions:

1. Spread butter on tortillas; place them in your air fryer's basket and cook them at 400 °F, for 3 minutes.

2. Meanwhile; in a bowl, mix tuna with zucchini, mayo and mustard and stir.

3. Divide this mix on each tortilla, top with cheese, roll tortillas; place them in your air fryer's basket again and cook them at 400 °F, for 4 minutes more. Serve for lunch.

Nutrition Values: Calories: 162; Fat: 4; Fiber: 8; Carbs: 9; Protein: 4

Summer Squash Fritters

Preparation Time: 17 Minutes

Servings: 4

Ingredients:

- 3 oz. cream cheese

- 1 egg; whisked

- 1/2 tsp. oregano; dried

- 1/3 cup carrot; grated

- 2/3 cup bread crumbs

- A pinch of salt and black pepper

- 1 yellow summer squash; grated

- 2 tbsp. olive oil

Directions:

1. In a bowl; mix cream cheese with salt, pepper, oregano, egg, breadcrumbs, carrot and squash and stir well.

2. Shape medium patties out of this mix and brush them with the oil.

3. Place squash patties in your air fryer and cook them at 400 °F, for 7 minutes. Serve them for lunch.

Nutrition Values: Calories: 200; Fat: 4; Fiber: 7; Carbs: 8; Protein: 6

Asian Chicken

Preparation Time: 40 Minutes

Servings: 4

Ingredients:

- 2 chicken breasts; skinless, boneless and sliced
- 1 tsp. olive oil
- 1 yellow onion; sliced
- 1 tbsp. Worcestershire sauce
- 14 oz. pizza dough
- 1 ½ cups cheddar cheese; grated
- 1/2 cup jarred cheese sauce
- Salt and black pepper to the taste

Directions:

1. Preheat your air fryer at 400 degrees F; add half of the oil and onions and fry them for 8 minutes, stirring once.

2. Add chicken pieces, Worcestershire sauce, salt and pepper; toss, air fry for 8 minutes

more, stirring once and transfer everything to a bowl.

3. Roll pizza dough on a working surface and shape a rectangle.

4. Spread half of the cheese all over, add chicken and onion mix and top with cheese sauce.

5. Roll your dough and shape into a U.

6. Place your roll in your air fryer's basket, brush with the rest of the oil and cook at 370 degrees for 12 minutes, flipping the roll halfway. Slice your roll when it's warm and serve for lunch.

Nutrition Values: Calories: 300; Fat: 8; Fiber: 17; Carbs: 20; Protein: 6

Parmesan Gnocchi

Preparation Time: 27 Minutes

Servings: 4

Ingredients:

- 1/4 cup parmesan; grated
- 1 yellow onion; chopped
- 16 oz. gnocchi
- 1 tbsp. olive oil
- 3 garlic cloves; minced
- 8 oz. spinach pesto

Directions:

1. Grease your air fryer's pan with olive oil, add gnocchi, onion and garlic, toss; put pan in your air fryer and cook at 400 °F, for 10 minutes.

2. Add pesto, toss and cook for 7 minutes more at 350 degrees F. Divide among plates and serve for lunch.

Nutrition Values: Calories: 200; Fat: 4; Fiber: 4; Carbs: 12; Protein: 4

Prosciutto Sandwich

Preparation Time: 15 Minutes

Servings: 1

Ingredients:

- 2 bread slices
- 2 prosciutto slices
- 2 basil leaves
- 1 tsp. olive oil
- 2 mozzarella slices
- 2 tomato slices
- A pinch of salt and black pepper

Directions:

1. Arrange mozzarella and prosciutto on a bread slice.

2. Season with salt and pepper; place in your air fryer and cook at 400 °F, for 5 minutes. Drizzle oil over prosciutto, add tomato and basil; cover with the other bread slice, cut sandwich in half and serve.

Nutrition Values: Calories: 172; Fat: 3; Fiber: 7; Carbs: 9; Protein: 5

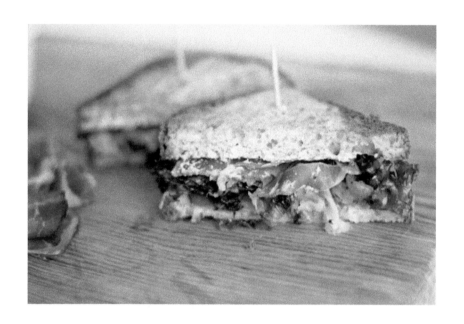

Chinese Style Pork

Preparation Time: 22 Minutes

Servings: 4

Ingredients:

- 2 lbs. pork; cut into medium cubes
- 2 eggs
- 1 cup cornstarch
- 1 tsp. sesame oil
- A pinch of Chinese five spice
- 3 tbsp. canola oil
- Sweet tomato sauce for serving
- Salt and black pepper to the taste

Directions:

1. In a bowl; mix five spice with salt, pepper and cornstarch and stir.

2. In another bowl; mix eggs with sesame oil and whisk well.

3. Dredge pork cubes in cornstarch mix; then dip in eggs mix and place them in your air fryer which you've greased with the canola oil.

4. Cook at 340 °F, for 12 minutes; shaking the fryer once. Serve pork for lunch with the sweet tomato sauce on the side.

Nutrition Values: Calories: 320; Fat: 8; Fiber: 12; Carbs: 20; Protein: 5

Fish And Kettle Chips

Preparation Time: 22 Minutes

Servings: 2

Ingredients:

- 2 medium cod fillets; skinless and boneless
- 1/4 cup buttermilk
- 3 cups kettle chips; cooked
- Salt and black pepper to the taste

Directions:

1. In a bowl mix fish with salt, pepper and buttermilk; toss and leave aside for 5 minutes.

2. Put chips in your food processor, crush them and spread them on a plate.

3. Add fish and press well on all sides.

4. Transfer fish to your air fryer's basket and cook at 400 °F, for 12 minutes. Serve hot for lunch.

Nutrition Values: Calories: 271; Fat: 7; Fiber: 9; Carbs: 14; Protein: 4

Egg Rolls

Preparation Time: 25 Minutes

Servings: 4

Ingredients:

- 1/2 cup mushrooms; chopped.
- 1/2 cup carrots; grated
- 1/2 cup zucchini; grated
- 8 egg roll wrappers
- 1 eggs; whisked
- 2 green onions; chopped.
- 2 tbsp. soy sauce
- 1 tbsp. cornstarch

Directions:

1. In a bowl; mix carrots with mushrooms, zucchini, green onions and soy sauce and stir well.

2. Arrange egg roll wrappers on a working surface; divide veggie mix on each and roll well.

3. In a bowl; mix cornstarch with egg, whisk well and brush eggs rolls with this mix.

4. Seal edges, place all rolls in your preheated air fryer and cook them at 370 °F, for 15 minutes. Arrange them on a platter and serve them for lunch.

Nutrition Values: Calories: 172; Fat: 6; Fiber: 6; Carbs: 8; Protein: 7

Special Pancake

Preparation Time: 20 Minutes

Servings: 2

Ingredients:

- 1 cup small shrimp; peeled and deveined
- 1 tbsp. butter
- 3 eggs; whisked
- 1/2 cup flour
- 1/2 cup milk
- 1 cup salsa

Directions:

1. Preheat your air fryer at 400 degrees F; add fryer's pan, add 1 tbsp. butter and melt it.

2. In a bowl; mix eggs with flour and milk, whisk well and pour into air fryer's pan, spread, cook at 350 degrees for 12 minutes and transfer to a plate. In a bowl; mix shrimp with salsa; stir and serve your pancake with this on the side.

Nutrition Values: Calories: 200; Fat: 6; Fiber: 8; Carbs: 12; Protein: 4

Turkish Style Koftas

Preparation Time: 25 Minutes

Servings: 2

Ingredients:

- 2 tbsp. feta cheese; crumbled
- 1 leek; chopped
- 1 tbsp. parsley; chopped
- 1 tsp. garlic; minced
- 1/2 lb. lean beef; minced
- 1 tbsp. cumin; ground
- 1 tbsp. mint; chopped
- Salt and black pepper to the taste

Directions:

1. In a bowl; mix beef with leek, cheese, cumin, mint, parsley, garlic, salt and pepper; stir well, shape your koftas and place them on sticks.

2. Add koftas to your preheated air fryer at 360 °F and cook them for 15 minutes. Serve them with a side salad for lunch.

Nutrition Values: Calories: 281; Fat: 7; Fiber: 8; Carbs: 17; Protein: 6

Chicken Wings

Preparation Time: 55 Minutes

Servings: 4

Ingredients:

- 3 lbs. chicken wings
- 3/4 cup potato starch
- 1 tsp. lemon juice
- 1/2 cup butter
- 1 tbsp. old bay seasoning
- Lemon wedges for serving

Directions:

1. In a bowl; mix starch with old bay seasoning and chicken wings and toss well.

2. Place chicken wings in your air fryer's basket and cook them at 360 °F, for 35 minutes shaking the fryer from time to time.

3. Increase temperature to 400 degrees F; cook chicken wings for 10 minutes more and divide them on plates.

4. Heat up a pan over medium heat; add butter and melt it.

5. Add lemon juice; stir well, take off heat and drizzle over chicken wings. Serve them for lunch with lemon wedges on the side.

Nutrition Values: Calories: 271; Fat: 6; Fiber: 8; Carbs: 18; Protein: 18

Summer Squash Fritters

Preparation Time: 17 Minutes

Servings: 4

Ingredients:

- 3 oz. cream cheese
- 1 egg; whisked
- 1/2 tsp. oregano; dried
- 1/3 cup carrot; grated
- 2/3 cup bread crumbs
- A pinch of salt and black pepper
- 1 yellow summer squash; grated
- 2 tbsp. olive oil

Directions:

1. In a bowl; mix cream cheese with salt, pepper, oregano, egg, breadcrumbs, carrot and squash and stir well.

2. Shape medium patties out of this mix and brush them with the oil.

3. Place squash patties in your air fryer and cook them at 400 °F, for 7 minutes. Serve them for lunch.

Nutrition Values: Calories: 200; Fat: 4; Fiber: 7; Carbs: 8; Protein: 6

Fresh Style Chicken

Preparation Time: 32 Minutes

Servings: 4

Ingredients:

- 2 chicken breasts; skinless, boneless and cubed
- 1/2 tsp. thyme; dried
- 10 oz. alfredo sauce
- 8 button mushrooms; sliced
- 1 red bell pepper; chopped
- 1 tbsp. olive oil
- 6 bread slices
- 2 tbsp. butter; soft

Directions:

1. In your air fryer, mix chicken with mushrooms, bell pepper and oil; toss to coat well and cook at 350 °F, for 15 minutes.

72

2. Transfer chicken mix to a bowl; add thyme and alfredo sauce, toss, return to air fryer and cook at 350 °F, for 4 minutes more.

3. Spread butter on bread slices; add it to the fryer, butter side up and cook for 4 minutes more. Arrange toasted bread slices on a platter; top each with chicken mix and serve for lunch.

Nutrition Values: Calories: 172; Fat: 4; Fiber: 9; Carbs: 12; Protein: 4

Greek Bar B Q
Sandwiches

Preparation Time: 13 minutes

Servings: 3

Ingredients:

- Barbecue sauce-1/3 cup
- Bacon slices-8 -cooked and cut into thirds
- Pita pockets-2 -halved
- Honey-2 tbsps
- Lettuce-1-1/4 cups -torn
- Red bell peppers-2 -sliced
- Tomatoes-2 -sliced

Directions:

1. Take a bowl and mix the barbecue sauce with honey.

2. After whisking finely, brush the bacon and bell peppers with this mixture.

3. Insert the bacon and bell peppers in your air fryer.

4. Cook at 350 o F for 6 minutes. During cooking shake once.

5. Fill the pita pockets with the bacon and bell peppers mixture.

6. Add some tomatoes and lettuce in the end.

7. To serve, garnish with the rest of the barbecue sauce and honey. Enjoy!

Nutrition Values:

calories 206, fat 6, fiber 9, carbs 14, protein 5

Unique Pie

Preparation Time: 22 minutes

Servings: 3

Ingredients:

- A large chicken breast -boneless, skinless and cubed
- Yellow onion-1 -chopped
- Soy sauce-1 tsp
- Salt and black pepper to taste
- Garlic powder-1/2 tsp
- White flour-1 tbsp
- Puff pastry sheets-2
- Carrot-1 -chopped
- White mushrooms-6 -chopped
- Italian seasoning-1 tsp
- Worcestershire sauce-1 tsp
- Milk-1 tbsp
- Olive oil-2 tbsps

Directions:

1. Warm up a pan with half of the oil over medium-high heat.

2. Mix the carrots with onions and stir.

3. Cook them for 2 minutes.

4. Add the chicken, mushrooms, salt, soy sauce, pepper, Italian seasoning, garlic powder, Worcestershire sauce, flour, and milk.

5. Mix them all really well and then remove from the heat.

6. Insert a puff pastry sheet on the bottom of your air fryer's pan.

7. Layer the chicken mix on it and top with another puff pastry sheet.

8. Oil the pastry with the rest of the oil finely.

9. Place the pan in the fryer to cook at 360 o F.

10. After 8 minutes of cooking, slice to serve and enjoy.

Nutrition Values:

calories 270, fat 5, fiber 7, carbs 14, protein 5

Pizza Like Rolls

Preparation Time: 43 minutes

Servings: 2

Ingredients:

- Olive oil-2 tsp
- Chicken breasts-2 -skinless, boneless and sliced
- Worcestershire sauce-1 tbsp
- Parmesan cheese-1-1/2 cups -grated
- Pizza dough-14 ounces
- Yellow onion-1 -sliced
- Tomato sauce-1/2 cup
- Salt and black pepper to taste

Directions:

1. Prepare your air fryer at 400 o F.

2. Throw in the onion and half of the olive oil in it to fry.

3. Cook for 8 minutes, shaking the fryer halfway.

4. Combine the chicken, Worcestershire sauce, salt and pepper and toss.

5. Fry for 8 more minutes, stirring once, then shift to a bowl.

6. On a working surface, roll the pizza dough and shape into a rectangle.

7. All over the dough, spread the cheese and then the chicken and onion mixture.

8. In the end, layer the tomato sauce to roll the dough.

9. Insert it in your air fryer's basket and brush the roll with the rest of the oil.

10. At 370 o F, cook for 14 minutes, flipping the roll halfway.

11. To serve, slice your roll.

Nutrition Values:

calories 270, fat 8, fiber 17, carbs 16, protein 6

Chinese Lunch

Preparation Time: 19 minutes

Servings: 5

Ingredients:

- Eggs-2

- Cornstarch-1 cup

- Chinese five spice-1/4 tsp

- Pork stew meat-2 pounds -cubed

- Salt and black pepper to taste

- Olive oil-3 tbsps

- Sesame oil-1 tsp

Directions:

1. Pick a bowl finely mix the Chinese spice, salt, pepper, and cornstarch.

2. Take another bowl to whisk the eggs and sesame oil very well.

3. Fold the pork cubes in the cornstarch mixture and then dip them in the egg mix.

4. Keep the pork cubes in your air fryer and then drizzle all over with the olive oil.

5. Cook at 360 o F for 12 minutes.

6. Share into the serving bowls with a side salad

Nutrition Values:

calories 270, fat 8, fiber 12, carbs 16, protein 5

Wings in Old Bay Style

Preparation Time: 52 minutes

Servings: 3

Ingredients:

- Chicken wings-3 pounds
- Old Bay seasoning-1 tbsp
- Lemon juice-1 tsp
- Butter-1/2 cup -melted
- Potato starch-3/4 cup

Directions:

1. Pick up a bowl and mix the chicken wings with the starch and Old Bay seasoning.

2. Toss the mixture well once again and then place the pieces in your air fryer's basket.

3. Prepare at 360 o F for 35 minutes, shaking the fryer from time to time.

4. Raise the temperature to 400 o F while frying the chicken wings for 10 more minutes.

5. Present the wings between plates to serve.

6. Top with the melted butter mixed with the lemon juice drizzled all over.

Nutrition Values:

calories 261, fat 6, fiber 8, carbs 18, protein 13

Dijon Special Hot Dogs

Preparation Time: 15 minutes

Servings: 3

Ingredients:

- Hot dog buns-3

- Dijon mustard-1 tbsp

- Hot dogs-3

- Parmesan cheese-2 tbsps -grated

Directions:

1. Put the hot dogs in preheated air fryer to cook at 390 o F for 5 minutes.

2. Add the hot dogs into the buns.

3. Spread the mustard all over, and sprinkle with the Parmesan.

4. Fry the hot dogs at 390 o F for 3 more minutes.

5. Serve and enjoy!

Nutrition Values:

calories 251, fat 7, fiber 8, carbs 16, protein 7

Lentil Cake Bites

Preparation Time: 22minutes

Servings: 2

Ingredients:

- Canned yellow lentils-1 cup -drained
- Turmeric powder-1/2 tsp
- Hot chili pepper-1 -chopped
- Garam masala-1 tsp
- Ginger-1 tsp -grated
- Baking powder-1 tsp
- Olive oil-2 tsp
- Water-1/3 cup water
- Salt and black pepper to taste
- Cilantro-1/2 cup -chopped
- Garlic cloves-4 -minced
- Baby spinach-1-1/2 cups -chopped
- Yellow onion-3/4 cup -chopped

Directions:

1. Bring your blender and add all ingredients in it.

2. Blend the mixture very well and then shape into two medium cakes.

3. Keep the lentils cakes in your preheated air fryer at 400 o F.

4. Let it cook for 10 minutes. Leave for few seconds.

5. Serve the lentil cakes on plates and enjoy.

Nutrition Values:

calories 182, fat 2, fiber 8, carbs 16, protein 4

Beefy Balls with Sauce

Preparation Time: 27 minutes

Servings: 3

Ingredients:

- Lean ground beef-1 pound
- Garlic cloves-2 -minced
- Panko breadcrumbs-1/4 cup
- Salt and black pepper to taste
- An egg yolk
- Olive oil-1 tbsp
- Red onion-1 -chopped
- Tomato sauce-16 ounces

Directions:

1. Pick a bowl and mix all the ingredients except for the tomato sauce and olive oil.

2. Mix well and then shape into medium-sized meatballs.

3. Oil the meatballs evenly and place them in your air fryer.

4. Cook at 400 o F for 10 minutes.

5. Warm up a pan over medium heat and pour the tomato sauce.

6. Heat it up for 2 minutes and then insert the meatballs.

7. Toss them a bit, and cook for 3 more minutes.

8. Dish out evenly the meatballs between plates and serve to eat.

Nutrition Values:

calories 270, fat 8, fiber 9, carbs 16, protein 4

Meatball Sandwiches

Preparation Time: 34 minutes

Servings: 3

Ingredients:

- Baguettes-3 -sliced halfway
- Tomato sauce-7 ounces
- Egg-1 -whisked
- Parmesan cheese-2 tbsps -grated
- Olive oil-1 tbsp
- Fresh basil-1 tsp -chopped
- Beef-14 ounces -minced
- Yellow onion-1 -chopped
- Breadcrumbs-1 tbsp
- Oregano-1 tbsp -chopped
- Salt and black pepper to taste

Directions:

1. Take a bowl to mix all ingredients except the tomato sauce, oil, and baguettes.

2. After stirring well, shape into medium-sized meatballs.

3. Warm up your air fryer with the oil at 375 o F to add the meatballs.

4. Prepare them for 12 minutes, flipping them halfway.

5. Pour the tomato sauce and cook for 10 more minutes.

6. Dish out the meatballs with sauce on half of the baguette halves.

7. Finally top with the other baguette halves to serve.

Nutrition Values:

calories 280, fat 9, fiber 6, carbs 16, protein 15

Kale Salad with Cod Fillets

Preparation Time: 22minutes

Servings: 2

Ingredients:

- Black cod fillets-2 -boneless
- Salt and black pepper to taste
- Grapes-1 cup -halved
- Pecans-1/2 cup
- Olive oil-2 tbsps + 1 tsp
- A fennel bulb -thinly sliced
- Kale leaves-3 cups -shredded
- Balsamic vinegar-2 tsp

Directions:

1. Season the fish with salt and pepper to place the fish in your air fryer's basket.

2. Drizzle a tsp of the olive oil over the fish to cook at 400 o F for 10 minutes.

3. Divide fish between plates.

4. Pick a bowl to mix the fennel, grapes, kale, pecans, vinegar, and 2 tbsps of oil.

5. After fine tossing, dish out.

6. Serve the salad next to the fish and enjoy.

Nutrition Values:

calories 240, fat 4, fiber 2, carbs 15, protein 12

Simple Turkey Dish

Preparation Time: 1 hour and 13 minutes

Servings: 7

Ingredients:

- Whole turkey breast-1

- Sweet paprika-1/2 tsp

- Salt and black pepper to taste

- Mustard-2 tbsps

- Olive oil-2 tsp

- Thyme-1 tsp -dried

- Butter-1 tbsp -melted

- Maple syrup-1/4 cup

Directions:

1. Use oil to brush over the turkey breast.

2. Marinate salt, pepper, paprika, and thyme and rub the seasoning well into the turkey breast.

3. Keep the turkey in your air fryer and cook at 350 o F for 25 minutes.

4. Turn the turkey breast and cook for 12 minutes more.

5. Again change the side and cook for another 12 minutes.

6. Take a bowl to whisk the butter, mustard, and maple syrup very well.

7. Brush the turkey breast with the maple syrup mixture.

8. Leave to cook for another 5 minutes.

9. Shift the meat to a cutting board and slice.

10. If desired, serve with a side salad.

Nutrition Values:

calories 230, fat 13, fiber 3, carbs 16, protein 11

Cod Balls Lunch

Preparation Time: 24 minutes

Servings: 5

Ingredients:

- Fresh cilantro-3 tbsps -minced

- Yellow onion-1 -chopped

- Salt and black pepper to taste

- Garlic cloves-2 -minced

- Panko breadcrumbs-1/4 cup

- Cod-1 pound -skinless and chopped

- Egg-1

- Sweet paprika-1/2 tsp

- Oregano-1/2 tsp -ground

- A drizzle of olive oil

Directions:

1. Pick your food processor and clean to mix all ingredients except the oil.

2. After blending well, shape medium-sized meatballs out of this mix.

3. Insert the meatballs in your air fryer's basket.

4. Let them grease with oil, and cook at 320 o F for 12 minutes, shaking halfway.

5. Divide the meatballs between plates and, if desired, serve with a side salad.

Nutrition Values:

calories 230, fat 9, fiber 3, carbs 10, protein 15

Stew-Potato & Beef

Preparation Time: 37 minutes

Servings: 5

Ingredients:

- Beef stew meat-2 pounds -cubed

- Gold potatoes-4 -cubed

- Beef stock-1 quart

- A handful of cilantro -chopped

- Carrot-1 -sliced

- Salt and black pepper to taste

- Smoked paprika-1/2 tsp

- Worcestershire sauce-4 tbsps

Directions:

1. Take a pan that fits your air fryer; mix all the ingredients well except the cilantro.

2. Keep it in your air fryer to cook at 375 o F.

3. After 25 minutes, divide into bowls.

4. Sprinkle the cilantro on top. Serve right away.

Nutrition Values:

calories 250, fat 8, fiber 1, carbs 20, protein 17

Pasta With Shrimp

Preparation Time: 27 minutes

Servings: 5

Ingredients:

- Spaghetti-5 ounces -cooked
- Salt and black pepper to taste
- Butter-1 tbsp -melted
- Shrimp-8 ounces -peeled and de veined
- Garlic cloves-5 -minced
- Chili powder-1 tsp
- Olive oil-2 tbsp

Directions:

1. Add 1 tbsp of the oil, along with the butter, in your air fryer.

2. Preheat the air fryer at 350 o F and add the shrimp.

3. Cook for 10 minutes and then combine all other ingredients, including the remaining a tbsp of oil,

4. Toss and cook for 5 minutes more.

5. Divide between plates, serve, and enjoy.

Nutrition Values:

calories 270, fat 7, fiber 4, carbs 15, protein 6

Ravioli Lunch Meal

Preparation Time: 12minutes

Servings: 5

Ingredients:

- Cheese ravioli-15 ounces

- Butter-1 tsp -melted

- Breadcrumbs-2 cups

- Buttermilk-1 cup

- Marinara sauce-10 ounces

- Cheddar cheese-1/4 cup -grated

Directions:

1. Pour the buttermilk in one bowl and add the breadcrumbs in another.

2. In buttermilk, dip ravioli, then in breadcrumbs.

3. Place the ravioli in your air fryer's basket and brush them with the melted butter.

4. Cook at 400 o F for 5 minutes and then divide the ravioli between plates.

5. Sprinkle the cheddar cheese on top, and serve.

Nutrition Values:

calories 260, fat 12, fiber 4, carbs 14, protein 11

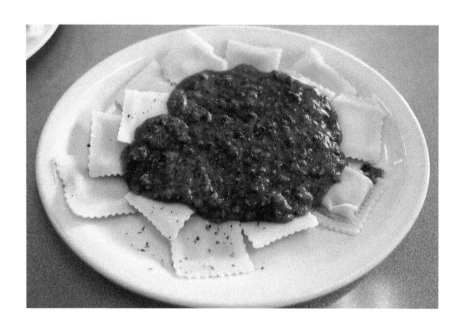

Curry Made With Cod

Preparation Time: 27 minutes

Servings: 5

Ingredients:

- Cod fillets-4 -skinless, boneless and cubed
- Curry paste-2 tsp
- Milk-1-1/2 cups -heated up
- Ginger-2 tsp -grated
- Cilantro-2 tbsps -chopped
- Salt and black pepper to taste

Directions:

1. Take a bowl and mix the milk, curry paste, ginger, salt, and pepper.

2. Place the fish in a pan that fits your air fryer, and then add the milk and curry mixture together.

3. After tossing the mixtures gently, place the pan in the fryer.

4. Cook at 400 o F for 15 minutes, shaking halfway.

5. Divide the curry into bowls, sprinkle the cilantro on top, and serve.

Nutrition Values:

calories 260, fat 8, fiber 3, carbs 13, protein 9

Special Casserole For Lunch

Preparation Time: 42 minutes

Servings: 7

Ingredients:

- Butter-2 tbsps -melted
- Cream cheese-12 ounces -softened
- Yogurt-1 cup
- Salt and black pepper to taste
- Curry powder-2 tsp
- Chicken meat-2 cups -cooked and cubed
- Scallions-4 -chopped
- Cilantro-1/4 cup -chopped
- Monterey jack cheese-6 ounces -grated
- Almonds-1/2 cup -sliced
- Chutney-1/2 cup

Directions:

1. Take a baking dish that fits your air fryer and add all ingredients except the Monterey jack cheese.

2. After mixing well, sprinkle the Monterey jack cheese all over chicken mixture.

3. Place the dish in your air fryer, and cook at 350 o F for 25 minutes.

4. Divide between plates and serve.

Nutrition Values:

calories 280, fat 10, fiber 2, carbs 24, protein 15

Creamy Potatoes Meal

Preparation Time: 29 minutes

Servings: 3

Ingredients:

- Gold potatoes-4 -cut into medium wedges

- Eggs-2

- Garlic powder-1 tsp

- Salt and black pepper to taste

- Sour cream-1/4 cup

- Sweet paprika-1-1/2 tsp

- Olive oil-1 tsp

- Cajun seasoning-1/2 tsp

Directions:

1. Pick a bowl and mix the eggs with the sour cream, paprika, garlic powder, Cajun seasoning, salt, and pepper.

2. After whisking well, take a pan that fits your air fryer.

3. Grease with the oil and arrange the potatoes on the bottom of the pan.

4. Spread the sour cream to mix all over.

5. Keep the pan in the fryer and cook at 370 o F for 17 minutes.

6. Divide between plates and serve.

Nutrition Values:

calories 290, fat 8, fiber 2, carbs 15, protein 7

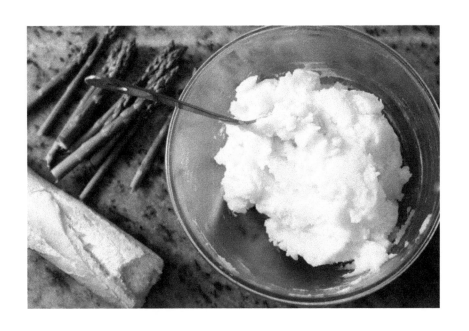

Lightning Source UK Ltd.
Milton Keynes UK
UKHW020634220621
385949UK00001B/59